ADHD DIET FOR KIDS

A Comprehensive Guide on Dietary Trick

for ADHD Kids with Recipes and Meal Plan

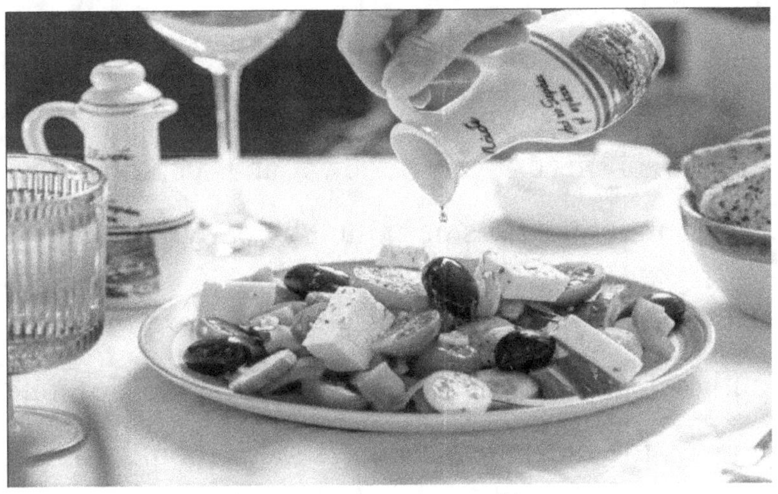

Elisa T. Morrison

Copyright © 2023 by Elisa T. Morrison

This book is a work of non-fiction. While the author has made every effort to provide accurate and up-to-date information, readers should consult with a professional in the relevant field before making any decisions based on the information in this book.

Table of Contents

INTRODUCTION

Millions of kids across the globe suffer from Attention Deficit Hyperactivity Disorder (ADHD), a neuro-developmental disease. It is characterized by signs including hyperactivity, impulsivity, and inattentiveness, which may make it challenging for kids to concentrate and finish activities.

A specific diet is one strategy for controlling the symptoms of ADHD. Some foods and nutrients have been shown in studies to help children with ADHD focus more, concentrate better, and have better general brain function. Foods that are rich in protein, healthy fats, and complex carbs are often included in a diet for ADHD.

These meals provide the brain with the nutrition it needs to work correctly while also assisting in controlling blood sugar levels, which can be a big problem for kids with ADHD.

Attention Deficit Hyperactivity Disorder has been identified in my younger brother, Alex. After conducting some study on the topic since our parents were concerned about how to assist him manage his illness, we learned about the ADHD diet.

The goal of the ADHD diet is to enhance children's concentration, mood, and behavior. It entails removing certain meals and replacing them with others that are rich in nutrients vital to brain health.

To assist Alex, we decided to try the ADHD diet. We began by getting rid of sugar, synthetic dyes, and preservatives from his diet. Instead, our parents concentrated on feeding him nutritious meals that were high in vitamins, minerals, and antioxidants.

Alex initially resisted the adjustments. He missed his sweet foods and cereals with vibrant colors.

Yet, after a few weeks, we saw a significant change in his behavior. He was less agitated, more focused, and less prone to mood changes.

We presented new meals and dishes that Alex liked and found intriguing to ease the transition. We increased the amount of fruits and vegetables in his meals, including broccoli, blueberries, and avocados. We also incorporated items high in protein, such as chicken, almonds, and eggs, which helped Alex's blood sugar levels stay stable and lessened his cravings.

The ADHD diet gradually merged into Alex's daily routine. Our parents were overjoyed with his growth since he seemed calmer and more focused than before. Our parents understood that by encouraging their kid to eat healthfully, they were promoting his entire well-being.

Alex was able to control his illness and have a happy, healthy childhood because of the ADHD diet. I also acquired enough expertise to manage children's ADHD diets. Alex discovered that food could be used as medication and that by making wise decisions, he might have a successful future.

It's important to remember that ADHD is a complicated illness with no one treatment that works for everyone. Yet, you'll discover in this book how to use dieting to cure your children's ADHD.

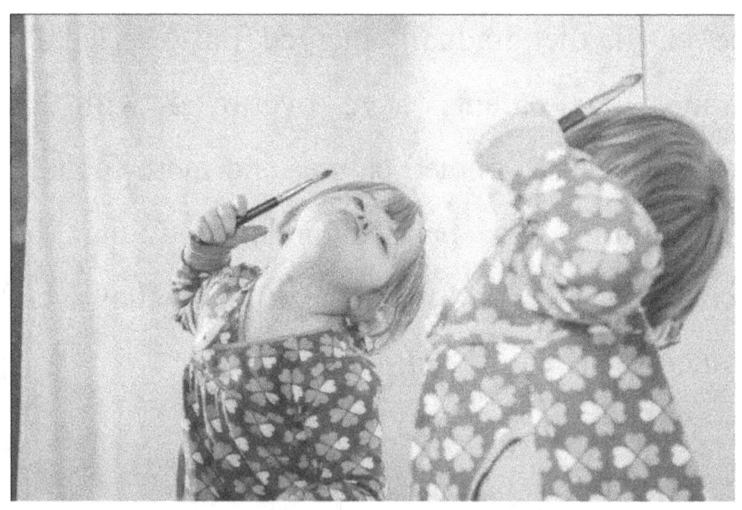

CHAPTER 1

What is ADHD in kids?

ADHD, commonly referred to as Attention Deficit Hyperactivity Disorder, is a neuro-developmental condition that impairs a child's capacity for focus, stillness, and impulse control. About 5–10% of kids worldwide are thought to have ADHD.

Inattention is one of the ADHD symptoms that stand out the most. Children with ADHD often struggle to maintain their attention on activities, carry out instructions, and organize their thoughts and possessions. Poor academic performance, forgetfulness, and disarray may result from this.

ADHD is also characterized by hyperactivity. Children that have this disease are often fidgety, extremely active, and unable to stay quiet for long periods. Moreover, they could speak excessively and regularly interrupt others.

Impulsivity is yet another essential trait of ADHD. Children with this disease often behave impulsively, which may result in actions like interrupting conversations, blurting out offensive remarks, and taking risks without thinking about the repercussions.

The social, intellectual, and emotional health of a kid may all be significantly impacted by ADHD. Making and keeping friendships, doing their schoolwork, and controlling their emotions may be difficult for kids with ADHD. They could also struggle with despair, anxiety, and poor self-esteem.

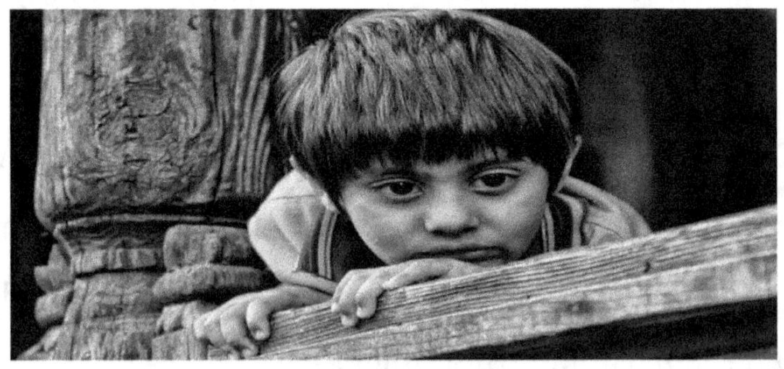

While the precise origins of ADHD are not fully known, evidence indicates that environmental and genetic factors may be involved.

According to some research, children with ADHD may not have enough dopamine or epinephrine in their brains.

Although there is no known therapy for ADHD, there are several approaches that may assist control symptoms. ADHD may be effectively managed with medication, behavioral therapy, lifestyle changes, and diets. A healthcare professional should be consulted by parents who believe their kid may have ADHD to get a precise diagnosis and create a unique treatment plan.

The intellectual, social, and emotional health of a kid may all be significantly impacted by ADHD. While there is no known therapy for this condition, there are powerful ones that may help control symptoms and enhance the quality of life. The greatest results for kids with ADHD depend on early diagnosis and treatment.

How Can Diet Affect ADHD Symptoms?

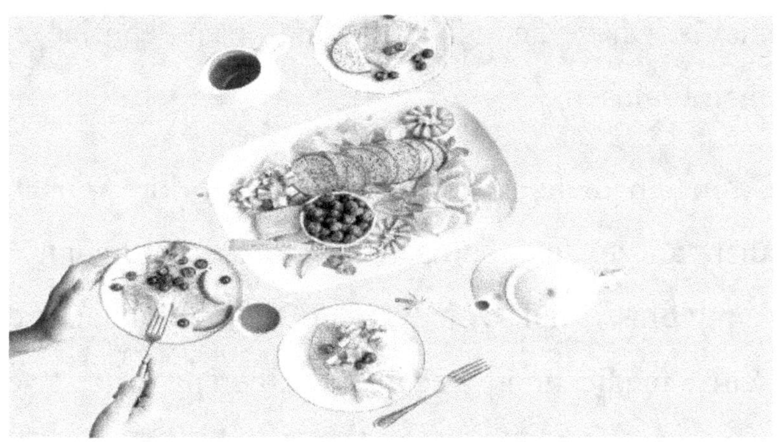

Impulsivity, inattention, and hyperactivity are traits of attention deficit hyperactivity disorder (ADHD). It may significantly disrupt interpersonal interactions as well as academic and professional performance in both children and adults.

Although there is no cure for ADHD, treating the symptoms with medication, counseling, and lifestyle changes may help people lead better lives. The effect of nutrition on ADHD symptoms is one such lifestyle change that has drawn more attention recently.

According to research, nutrition may significantly affect the symptoms of ADHD. Research has found that diets rich in sugar, processed, and glycemic index might exacerbate symptoms including hyperactivity and impulsivity.

On the other hand, it has been shown that a diet high in complete foods, such as fruits, vegetables, whole grains, and lean meats, may reduce the symptoms of ADHD.

Dopamine is a neurotransmitter that has been linked to how nutrition affects ADHD symptoms, according to one idea. A chemical messenger in the brain called dopamine aids in controlling mood, drive, and concentration. Dopamine levels in the brain are lower in those with ADHD, which may contribute to symptoms like impulsivity and inattentiveness.

Some meals, including those with a high glycemic index, may increase blood sugar levels quickly, which can affect the brain's dopamine levels. This may exacerbate the hyperactivity and impulsivity associated with ADHD symptoms.

Contrarily, meals high in vitamins and antioxidants, such as fruits and vegetables, may help control dopamine levels, enhancing mood and focusing. Studies have also shown that omega-3 fatty acids, which are included in seafood like salmon and tuna, might enhance cognitive performance and lessen ADHD symptoms.

There is evidence to support the notion that dietary habits may affect ADHD symptoms in addition to the effect of certain foods on those symptoms. For instance, it has been shown that a Mediterranean diet rich in whole foods, healthy fats, and plant-based proteins enhances cognitive performance and lessens ADHD symptoms. Similarly, it has been shown that eating a diet rich in protein and low in carbs will reduce the symptoms of ADHD.

There is mounting research that suggests food may significantly affect ADHD symptoms. Although more study is required to completely understand the relationship between nutrition and ADHD, people with ADHD are likely to benefit by adopting a nutritious diet high in whole foods, lean protein, and healthy fats.

Moreover, cutting down on processed meals, sweetened beverages, and other sources of empty calories may probably aid in symptom management and enhance the general quality of life.

The Role of Nutrition in ADHD Management

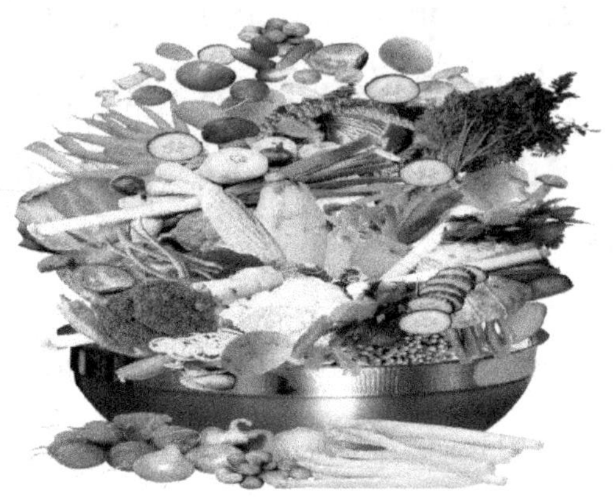

Although often diagnosed in children, ADHD may linger into adulthood. Nutritional therapies are becoming more popular as an alternative to or a supplement to medication as the most popular form of therapy for ADHD symptoms. As it gives the body the resources it needs to operate correctly, a good diet is vital to managing ADHD symptoms. It may either make them worse or make them go away.

Many studies have revealed a connection between the signs of ADHD and dietary deficits. Children with ADHD had reduced amounts of critical minerals including iron, zinc, magnesium, and omega-3 fatty acids, which are important for cognition, memory, mood management, and behavior, according to research in the Journal of Child Neurology.

Neurotransmitters are substances that convey messages in the brain, and deficiencies in certain nutrients might result in an imbalance of these chemicals.

Symptoms including inattention, impatience, and hyperactivity might result from this imbalance.

Polyunsaturated fats of the type omega-3 fatty acids are essential for the growth and operation of the brain. Many studies have shown that taking an omega-3 supplement may dramatically reduce the symptoms of ADHD. According to research in the Journal of Child Psychology and Psychiatry, children with ADHD who were given omega-3 supplements fared much better than those who got a placebo in terms of attention and hyperactivity.

Another research that appeared in the Journal of Developmental and Behavioral Pediatrics discovered that giving children with ADHD omega-3 supplements for six months greatly improved their attention, behavior, and cognitive ability.

Vitamin D, calcium, B vitamins, and iron are among the other vitamins and minerals that are lacking in people with ADHD. Studies have shown that children with ADHD had lower amounts of vitamin D compared to their peers, which is important for brain development.

Calcium has been demonstrated to have a soothing impact on people with ADHD and is essential for the healthy functioning of neurotransmitters. B vitamin supplementation may help children with ADHD pay attention and behave better, according to a meta-analysis of research on the subject.

Dopamine is a neurotransmitter that is necessary for motivation, mood, and attention, and iron is needed for its creation. Research has shown that iron supplementation help reduce the symptoms of ADHD in those who are iron deficient.

Also, reducing specific items from the diet helps lessen the effects of ADHD. According to research, food additives like artificial colors and preservatives might make some people's symptoms of ADHD worse. Artificial food coloring and preservatives were shown to make hyperactivity in children with ADHD worse, according to research published in The Lancet.

Reduced consumption of meals rich in sugar and refined carbs, according to another research in the Journal of Attention Disorders, reduced the symptoms of inattention in kids with ADHD.

To control the symptoms of ADHD, a proper diet is essential. The body can get the nutrients it needs via nutritional therapies, which may also help with ADHD symptoms.

ADHD symptoms have been shown to improve with omega-3 intake as well as vitamin and mineral supplements such as vitamin D, calcium, B vitamins, and iron. ADHD symptoms may also be reduced by cutting out certain items from the diet, such as those heavy in sugar, processed carbs, and artificial additives.

Nutritional treatments should be taken into consideration as a supplemental or alternative technique for controlling ADHD symptoms, even if medication is currently the most popular kind of therapy for the condition.

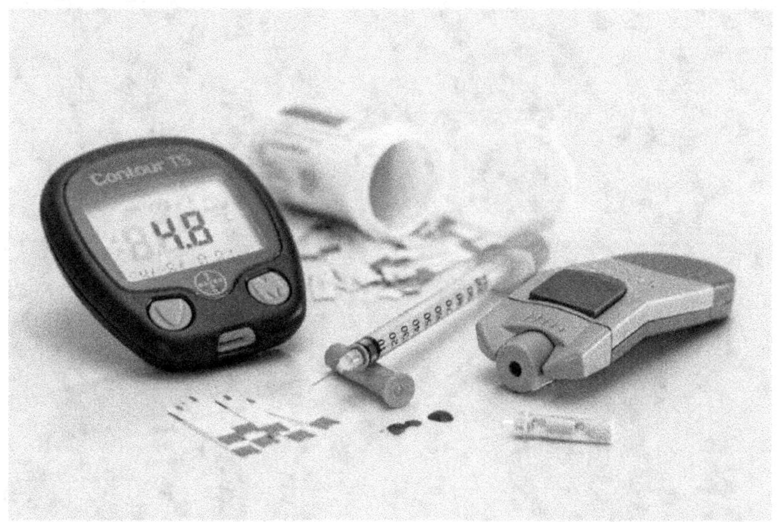

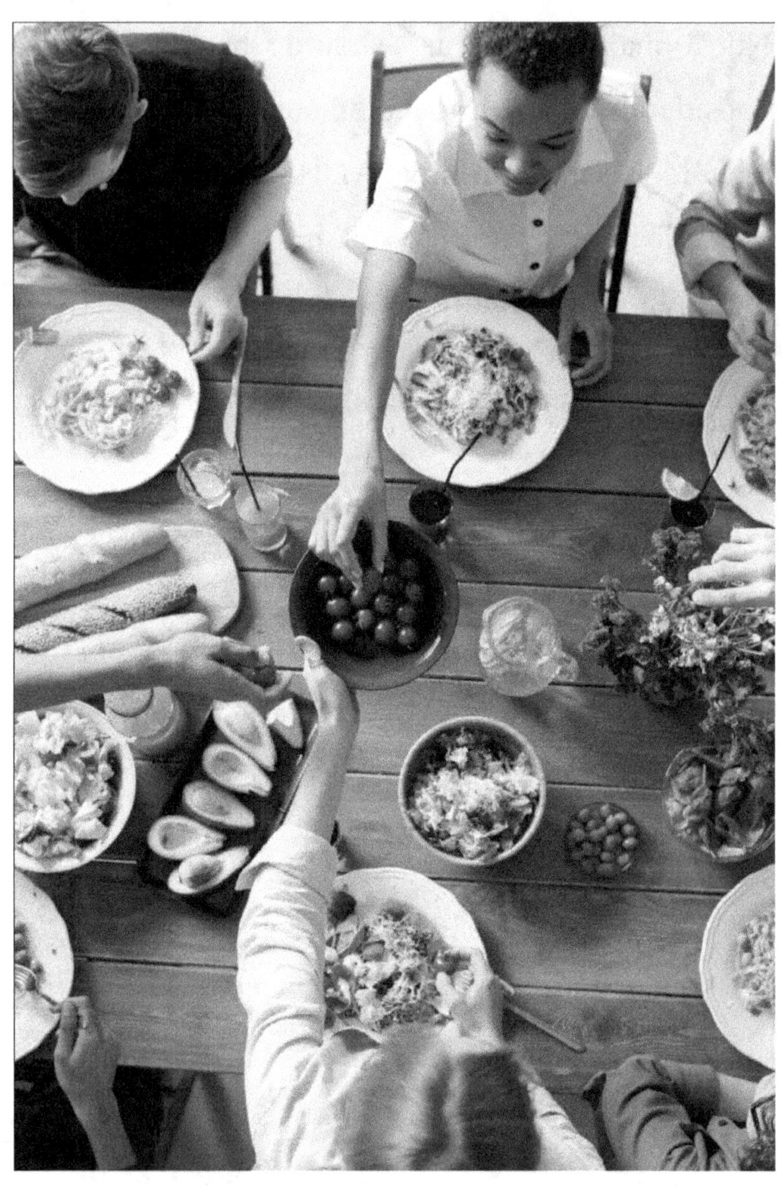

CHAPTER 2

Benefits of a Healthy Diet for Kids with ADHD

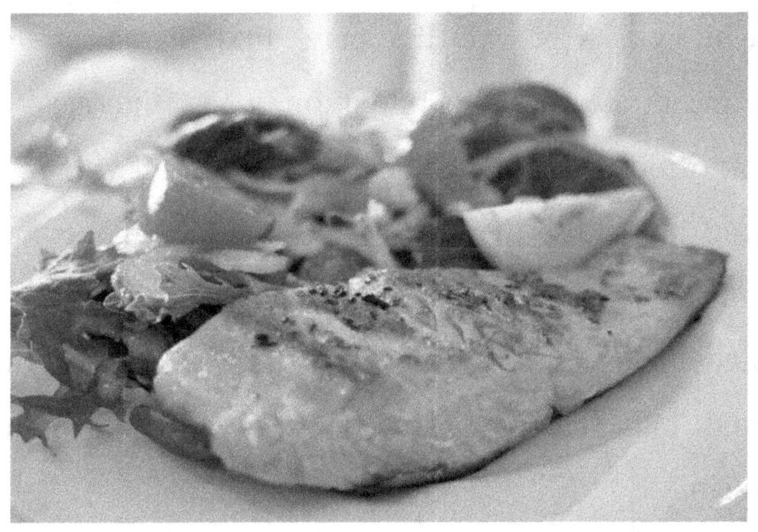

Maintaining a nutritious diet is just as important for treating ADHD as medication and behavioral treatment. A balanced mix of important nutrients is part of a healthy diet for children with ADHD, and specific items that might exacerbate the condition's symptoms should be avoided.

These are a few advantages of a balanced diet for children with ADHD.

1. Better Concentration and Attention

Children with ADHD may find it easier to concentrate and pay attention when they eat a nutritious diet that includes foods high in vitamins and minerals. It has been shown that certain nutrients, including omega-3 fatty acids, iron, zinc, and magnesium, are necessary for brain function and enhance memory, alertness, and attention span.

2. Decreased impulsivity and hyperactivity

Processed meals heavy in sodium, sugar, and artificial colorings and preservatives may make children's ADHD symptoms worse. Contrarily, a balanced diet low in sugar and processed foods may aid in lowering impulsivity and hyperactivity, making it simpler for kids to focus and regulate their behavior.

3. Improved Sleep Quality

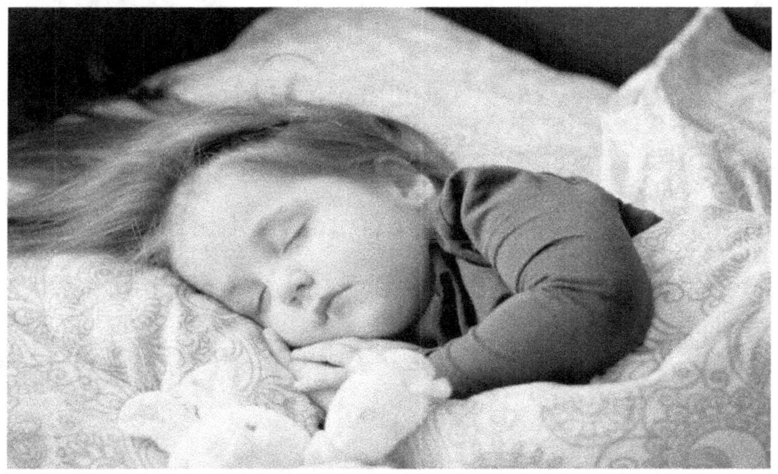

Having difficulties falling and staying asleep is a common sign of ADHD in children, which may make the symptoms worse. To help children with ADHD concentrate and pay attention throughout the day, a balanced diet that contains foods that promote sleep, such as whole grains, lean protein, and fresh fruits and vegetables, may enhance the quality of their nighttime sleep.

4. Increasing the Efficacy of Medicine

Children with ADHD often get prescriptions for medications like stimulants to help control their symptoms. Yet maintaining a healthy diet may also enhance the efficiency of prescription drugs. For instance, taking a drug with food that is heavy in fat might cause the medication's absorption to be slowed down and less effective. The efficacy of a drug, however, may be increased by taking it with a meal that includes protein and entire carbohydrates.

5. Health Has Improved Overall

For children with ADHD to grow and develop to their full potential, they need a balanced diet rich in whole foods, lean protein, fruits, and vegetables. Eating a healthy diet supports the immune system, which can help prevent illnesses that could exacerbate ADHD symptoms in children, helps them maintain a healthy weight, lowers their risk of developing other health conditions like diabetes and high blood pressure, and reduces the risk of other conditions like obesity.

A balanced diet is a crucial component in treating ADHD in kids. A healthy diet may help children with ADHD concentrate better, lessen impulsivity and hyperactivity, get better sleep, help medications work better, and generally enhance their health.

Working with a qualified dietitian as a parent may help you make sure your kid is eating a balanced diet that is suited to their requirements.

Perusing the Basics of a Healthy ADHD Diet

The basics of a healthy ADHD diet include:

1. Maintaining a healthy diet

For general health and well-being, a balanced diet made up of a range of whole foods is crucial. Lean protein, healthy fats, and a diet high in fruits, vegetables, and whole grains may boost brain health and lower inflammation. It is advised to follow a diet reduced in processed foods, sugar, and artificial additives.

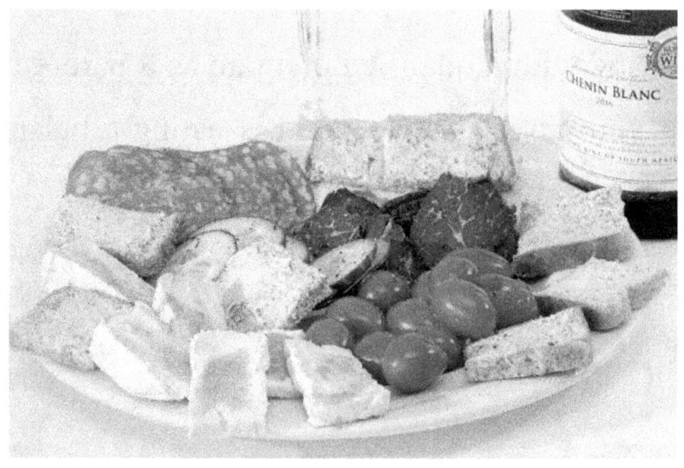

2. Ensuring an appropriate intake of protein

Protein is a necessary food that is critical to brain health. Consuming meals high in protein, such as chicken, fish, beans, and eggs, may aid with mood regulation, attention improvement, and maintaining energy throughout the day. Every meal should include protein, but breakfast is particularly important to help you get your day started.

3. Consuming Beneficial Fats

Omega-3 fatty acids are good fats that may help decrease inflammation and are crucial for brain function. Foods like avocado, salmon, nuts, seeds, and other healthy fats may enhance brain function and lessen the effects of ADHD.

4. Avoiding Allergies to Food

Inflammation and altered brain function may result from food allergies and sensitivities. Working with a healthcare professional is advised to recognize and prevent any dietary allergies or sensitivities.

5. Drinking water

Drinking enough water is crucial for general health and brain function. Water consumption may aid with attention, and mood regulation, and prevent dehydration, which can make ADHD symptoms worse.

6. Avoiding much sugar and caffeine

By boosting hyperactivity and impulsivity, caffeine and excessive sugar consumption may exacerbate ADHD symptoms. It is advised to minimize or stay away from sugary meals and beverages, as well as caffeinated drinks like soda and coffee.

A healthy ADHD diet should focus on getting enough protein and good fats, avoiding dietary allergies, keeping hydrated, and reducing caffeine and excess sugar. Working with a healthcare professional is vital to guarantee optimal nutrition and keep an eye out for any possible drug or other treatment interactions, just as with other dietary changes.

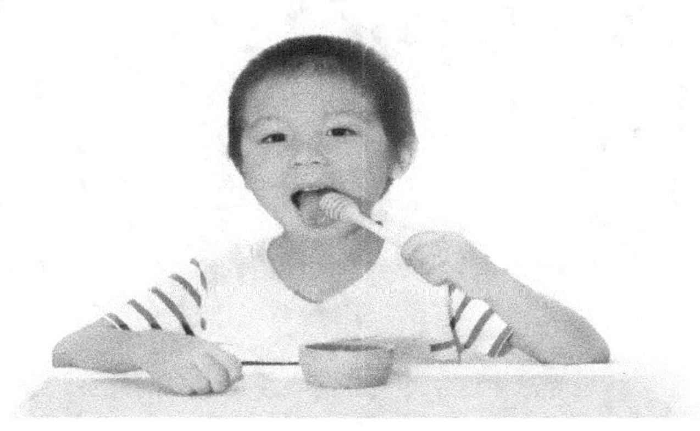

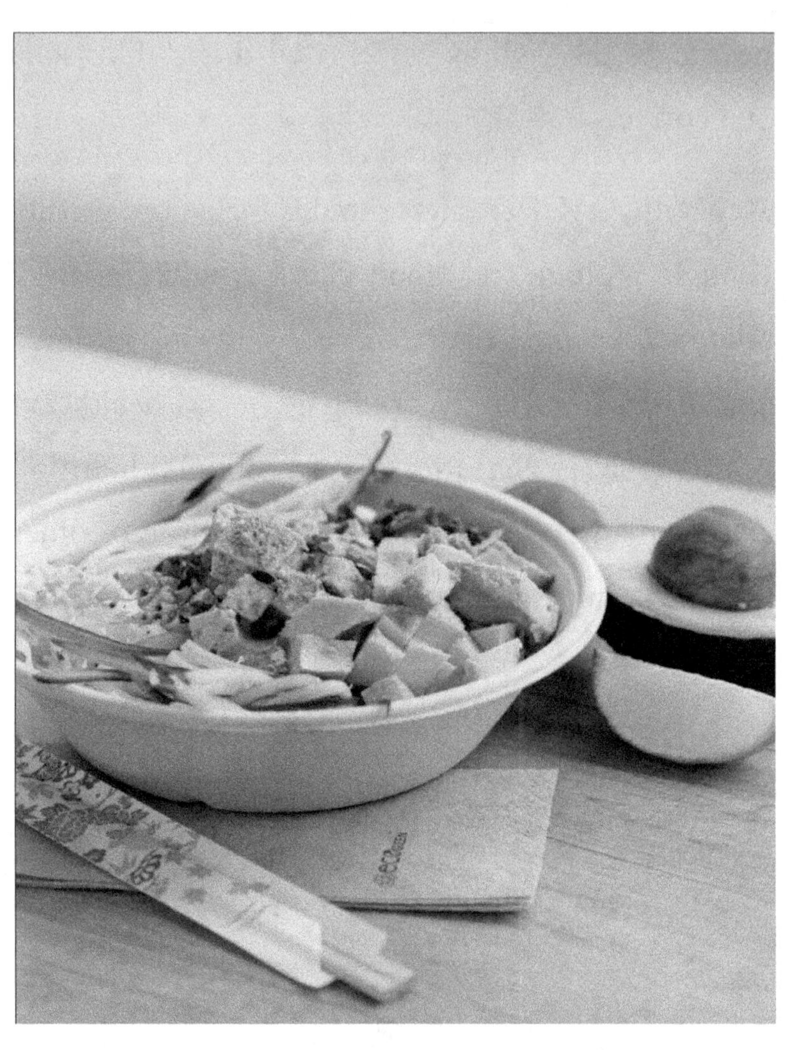

CHAPTER 3

ADHD Diet for Kids

Foods to Include In Kids' ADHD Diet

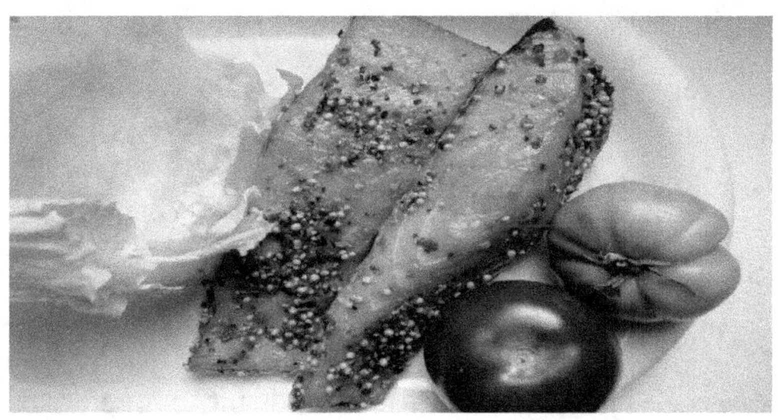

Children's hyperactivity, focus, and mood may all be impacted by certain diets. We will look at some of the foods that children with ADHD should eat in this book.

1. Fatty acids omega-3

The body is unable to manufacture the critical lipids known as omega-3 fatty acids. They are present in seeds, nuts, and fish. Omega-3 fatty acids are essential for brain growth and function, according to research. They may elevate mood, increase cognition, and lower inflammation. Children's ADHD symptoms have also been proven to be improved by omega-3 fatty acids.

2. Various Carbohydrates

Slow-releasing sugars known as complex carbs provide the brain with a consistent supply of energy. They may be found in fruits, vegetables, and whole grains. Complex carbohydrate foods are crucial for ADHD kids because they help control blood sugar levels, which helps lessen hyperactivity and impulsive behavior.

3. Protein

The building blocks of the body are proteins, which are required for tissue growth and repair. Also essential to brain health is protein. Lean meat, fish, eggs, and beans are examples of foods rich in protein that may assist to lessen the symptoms of ADHD. Blood sugar levels are stabilized by protein, which may lessen impulsivity and increase focus.

4. Iron

The growth and operation of the brain depend on iron, a vital element. Iron aids in the transport of oxygen, which the brain needs for maximum performance. Lean meat, eggs, and dark leafy greens are examples of foods strong in iron that may help to lessen the symptoms of ADHD.

5. Zinc

The mineral zinc is crucial for the growth and operation of the brain. Children with ADHD had lower zinc levels than those without ADHD, according to studies. Zinc-rich foods, such as oysters, lean meat, and pumpkin seeds, may assist to lessen the symptoms of ADHD.

6. B vitamin

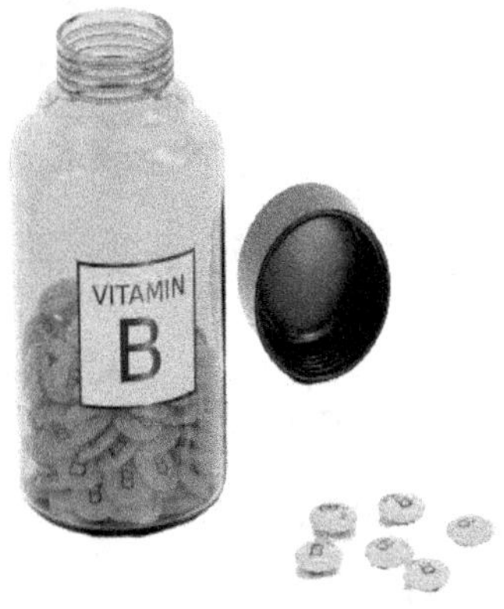

A set of vitamins known as vitamin B are crucial for the growth and operation of the brain. The efficient functioning of the brain requires the conversion of food into energy, which vitamin B aids with. Lean meat, healthy grains, and leafy greens are examples of foods strong in vitamin B that may help to lessen the symptoms of ADHD.

7. Water

For the brain to operate at its best, water is crucial. The focus and temperament of youngsters might be affected by dehydration. It is advised that kids consume a lot of water throughout the day.

Children's ADHD symptoms may be improved with a balanced diet that includes meals high in omega-3 fatty acids, complex carbohydrates, protein, iron, zinc, vitamin B, and water.

It is important to highlight that managing ADHD symptoms with food alone may not be sufficient. Children with ADHD should follow a complete treatment plan that includes food, medication, and behavioral therapy. To create a customized treatment plan, parents should speak with their child's doctor.

Foods to Avoid In Kids' ADHD Diet

Around 6-7% of school-aged children have Attention Deficit Hyperactivity Disorder (ADHD), a prevalent neurological condition. An appropriate ADHD diet should include nutritious food options devoid of processed foods, artificial colors, and chemicals.

It is commonly known that some foods, additives, or chemicals may make children's ADHD symptoms worse. The following foods should be avoided by kids with ADHD:

1. Finished Products:

Preservatives and artificial sweeteners are found in highly processed meals like packaged snacks and junk food. There is evidence that certain chemicals make children's ADHD symptoms worse. Moreover, processed meals are heavy in sugar and food chemicals, which might make kids more hyperactive and unfocused.

2. Sweet Foods

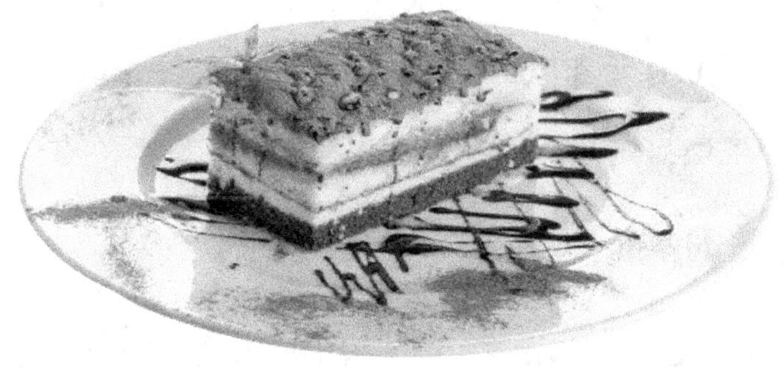

Some kids' symptoms of ADHD might become worse if they consume a lot of sugar. It has been shown that sugar makes kids more hyperactive, interferes with their sleep, and makes them moody. Sugar-sweetened beverages, candy, desserts, and other high-sugar meals should be avoided by kids with ADHD.

3. Preservatives and artificial food colors

Children's hyperactivity and symptoms of ADHD have been related to certain food additives, including artificial food colors (Red 40, Blue 1, and Yellow 5) and preservatives (BHA, BHT, and TBHQ). It is advised to stay away from processed meals that have these substances in them.

4. Casein and gluten

Some kids' symptoms of ADHD have been demonstrated to improve on a diet devoid of casein and gluten. Casein is a protein present in dairy products, while gluten is a protein found in wheat, barley, and rye. Foods containing casein and gluten should be avoided by children with ADHD, or they should transition to dairy- and gluten-free alternatives.

5. Salicylates:

Salicylates are organic substances that may be discovered in certain fruits, vegetables, and spices. Some ADHD kids may be sensitive to salicylates and may see their symptoms go worse after eating foods high in these chemicals. Fruits and vegetables such as berries, oranges, tomatoes, almonds, and cinnamon are high in salicylates.

6. Caffeine:

Children with ADHD may experience overstimulation, anxiety, and sleep issues as a result of caffeine. Caffeine-rich liquids, including coffee, tea, and energy drinks, should be avoided by kids with ADHD.

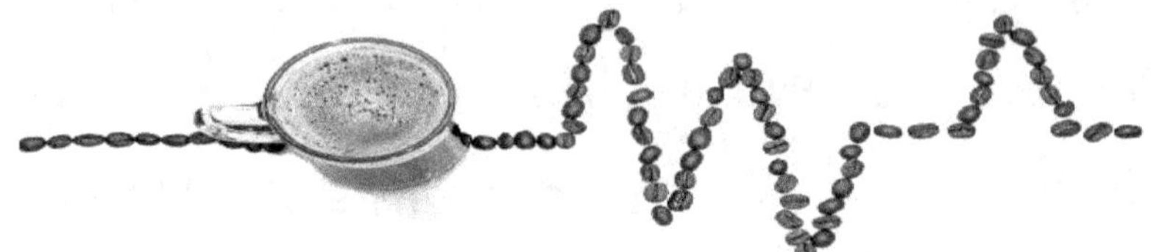

In conclusion, treating the symptoms of ADHD in youngsters may be greatly helped by a nutritious diet. Their diet should include foods that are minimally processed, devoid of chemical additives and artificial ingredients, and high in nutrients including lean protein, fruits, vegetables, and whole grains. Parents may assist their children in better managing their condition by avoiding foods that exacerbate the symptoms of ADHD.

CHAPTER 4

Tips for Meal Planning and Preparation

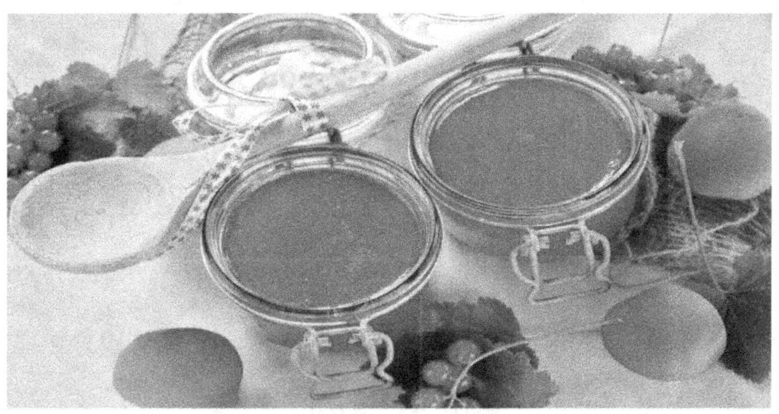

It can be difficult for a child with ADHD to maintain organization and attention during meals. Mealtimes don't have to be stressful, however, if a little amount of planning and preparation is done.

The following advice can help children with ADHD organize and prepare their meals:

1. Create a meal plan: Planning meals in advance may help ADHD children remain organized and avoid impulsive eating decisions. Plan your child's meals for the next week at a table together. Include a range of foods, such as whole grains, protein, veggies, and fruits.

2. Participate in grocery shopping with your kid: Taking your ADHD child with you to the supermarket will help them comprehend where food originates from and increase their interest in mealtime. Invite them to assist you with ingredient selection and nutrition label reading.

3. Employ visual aids: Images, checklists, and charts are all useful visual aids for children with ADHD. Make a chart listing the items your kid should consume at each meal and place it in a prominent location in the kitchen.

4. Keep things simple: Children with ADHD may find it stressful to prepare elaborate meals.

Concentrate on preparing fast, simple meals like stir-fries, salads, or sandwiches.

5. Plan: Making meals ahead of time may save time and ease stress related to mealtimes. Encourage your youngster to assist you in creating sandwiches or chopping veggies as you prepare meals and snacks in advance.

6. Promote awareness: Using mindfulness techniques while eating will help your kid with ADHD concentrate on their meals and avoid being sidetracked. Encourage children to chew their meals slowly and completely before taking a few calm, deep breaths.

7. Make it enjoyable: Mealtimes don't have to be dull! Encourage your youngster to use creativity while preparing meals, such as by creating colorful fruit kabobs or sprinkling pizza with extra ingredients. By doing this, they may find eating to be more interesting and pleasurable.

These guidelines may help youngsters with ADHD learn how to arrange their meal planning and preparation in a stress-free manner.

Not only does this keep children engaged throughout meals, but it may also encourage more healthful eating practices in general.

Meal Ideas and Recipes

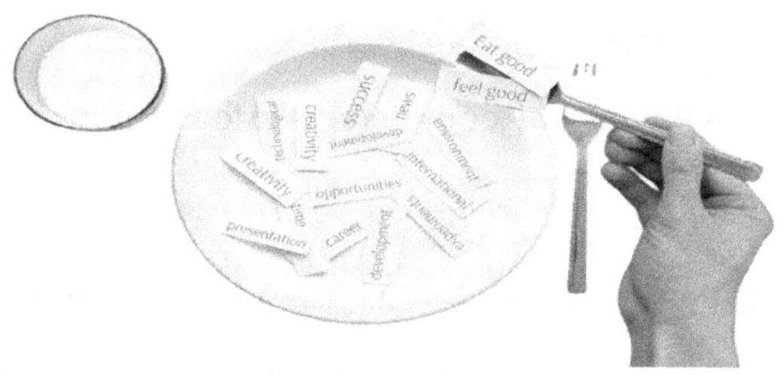

Millions of youngsters throughout the globe suffer from attention deficit hyperactivity disorder (ADHD). Although medicine and therapy are popular forms of treatment, food and nutrition may also be important in controlling symptoms. Giving your child balanced, nutrient-rich meals may enhance concentration, lessen impulsivity, and boost general well-being. Here are some recipes and meal suggestions to help youngsters with ADHD manage their symptoms:

Breakfast suggestions for ADHD children

1. Whole-wheat bread with scrambled eggs and spinach

2. Greek yogurt topped with granola and berries

3. Smoothie (banana, spinach, almond milk, and honey)

4. Oatmeal with sliced banana, almonds, and chia seeds

5. Sandwich on a whole-wheat English muffin with turkey, bacon, and cheese

Lunch Recipes for ADHD Children

1. Roll up Turkey and cheese together with cucumber slices and cherry tomatoes

2. A salad of grilled chicken with sliced almonds, berries, and mixed greens.

3. Whole-wheat pita filled with chopped chicken, hummus, and vegetables

4. Whole-grain bread with a tuna sandwich with carrot and celery sticks

5. Baked sweet potato topped with salsa, avocado, and black beans

CHAPTER 5

Recipes for Children with ADHD

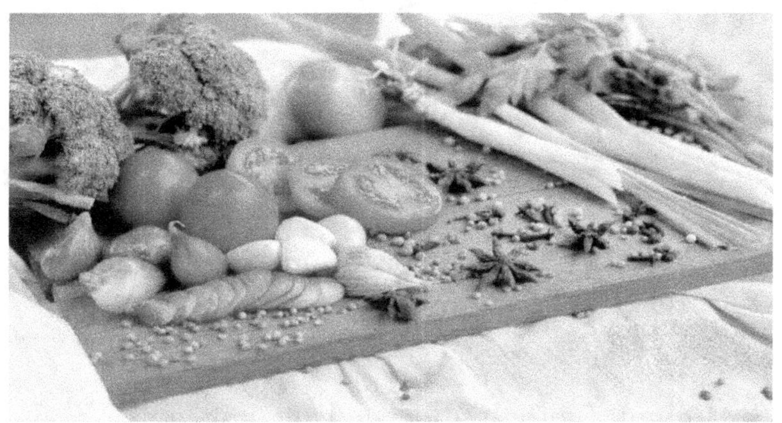

1. Broccoli and quinoa with baked salmon

2. Whole-wheat spaghetti served with zucchini and turkey meatballs

3. Stir-fried chicken with mixed vegetables, brown rice, and

4. Sweet potato wedges with slow-cooked jerked pork

5. Roasted carrots and brussels sprouts with baked chicken

Snacks:

1. Apple slices with almond or peanut butter as a snack.

2. Popcorn that has been air-popped and has nutritious yeast on top

3. Hummus with thinly sliced cucumbers

4. Whole-grain crackers and grapes with cheese

5. Carrot sticks with Greek yogurt ranch dip

Recipes and Instructions

1. Quinoa Stir-Fry Bowl:

Ingredients:

- 1 cup quinoa

- 1 tablespoon olive oil

- 1 onion, chopped

- 1 bell pepper, chopped

- 1 zucchini, chopped

- 2 garlic cloves, minced

- 1 tablespoon low-sodium soy sauce

- 1 teaspoon sesame oil

- 1 teaspoon honey

- Salt and pepper

Directions:

1. Wash the quinoa and cook accordingly.

2. Heat the olive oil with medium heat. Pour onion and make sure to cook for 2-3 minutes.

3. Add bell pepper, zucchini, and garlic to the skillet, and cook for another 5 minutes.

4. Add cooked quinoa to the skillet, along with soy sauce, sesame oil, and honey. Mix well.

5. Season with salt and pepper, and serve.

2. Baked sweet potato fries:

Ingredients:

- Two medium sweet potatoes, gently peeled and made into fries

- 1 tablespoon olive oil

- 1 teaspoon garlic powder

- 1 teaspoon smoked paprika

- Salt and pepper

Directions:

1. Preheat the oven to 400°F.

2. Toss sweet potato fries in olive oil and seasonings.

3. Place in a single layer on a baking sheet.

4. Bake for 20 to 25 minutes, or until golden and crispy.

3. Greek Yogurt Berry Smoothie:

Ingredients:

- 1 cup Greek yogurt

- A cup of mixed fresh or frozen berries

- 1 banana

- One tablespoon of honey

- ½ cup unsweetened almond milk

Directions:

1. Add all ingredients to a blender, and blend until smooth.

2. Pour into a glass and serve immediately.

Finally, feeding your kid balanced meals and snacks may help them control their symptoms of ADHD and enhance their general well-being.

It may also be advantageous to include whole meals that are high in nutrients while limiting processed foods and sweets. These menu suggestions and recipes are a great place to start, but for tailored nutrition advice, it's always important to speak with a healthcare provider.

Other Suggestions for Meal Ideas and Recipes

Youngsters with ADHD may exhibit signs of hyperactivity and often struggle to control their urges. Planning and preparing healthy meals for them might be challenging for parents because of their inability to concentrate for extended periods.

Here are some ideas for dishes and meals that parents may use to meet the particular dietary demands of their children:

1. High-protein breakfast: If a kid has ADHD, a high-protein breakfast may help them maintain a steady level of energy throughout the day. A fantastic way to start the day is with a breakfast burrito, scrambled eggs, whole-grain bread, or oatmeal.

2. Healthful snacks: Kids with ADHD must maintain stable blood sugar levels all day. Other suggestions for snacks are yogurt with berries, roasted chickpeas, carrot sticks with hummus, and apple slices with peanut butter.

3. Lunches high in protein: A lunch high in protein will assist the youngster feel satisfied and focused for the remainder of the school day. Examples include whole-grain sandwiches with turkey or chicken, quinoa salads with cheese and vegetables, and grilled chicken over brown rice.

4. Omega-3 fatty acid-rich meals: Omega-3 fatty acids are known to support cognitive performance and brain health, which may be advantageous for kids with ADHD. Omega-3 fatty acids may be found in foods like baked salmon, tuna salad, and grilled shrimp with vegetables and brown rice.

5. Foods strong in iron and zinc: Leafy greens, beans, seeds, nuts, and lean red meat are all sources of iron and zinc, two nutrients that are essential for cognitive function. Other suggestions are spinach and cheese omelets, black bean tacos, and chicken stir-fry with vegetables.

Last but not least, always make it colorful and enjoyable. Consider experimenting with colors and textures to add interest to the meals since kids like food that looks enticing. When trying to convince a picky eater to eat a nutritious meal, presentation, and ingenuity may be quite helpful.

7days Meal Plan For Kids with ADHD

Day 1 Plan

- Eggs scrambled with whole wheat bread and orange juice for breakfast.
- Snack: Hummus-topped carrot sticks
- For lunch, have grilled chicken breast with brown rice and steamed broccoli.
- Snack: Apple slices and string cheese
- Dinner will consist of baked salmon, roasted sweet potatoes, and mixed veggies.

Day 2 Plan

- Yogurt parfait with fresh berries and granola for breakfast
- Snack: Trail mix with raisins and a variety of nuts.

- Lunch consists of a turkey and cheese sandwich, baby carrots, and ranch dressing.

- Quinoa-topped beef and vegetable stir-fry for dinner

Day 3 Plan

- Banana pancakes with turkey bacon and orange slices for breakfast.

- Apple with almond butter as a snack

- Tuna salad, whole grain crackers, and cucumber slices for lunch

- Snack: Parmesan cheese-topped popcorn.

- The supper will be grilled chicken, roasted broccoli, and sweet potato mash.

Day 4 Plan

- For breakfast, serve grapefruit slices on bread spread with peanut butter.

- Greek yogurt with honey and cinnamon, as a snack

- Grilled cheese sandwich and tomato soup for lunch
- Snack: Rice cakes with blueberries and cream cheese
- For dinner, roast asparagus and wild rice with lemon-garlic shrimp.

Day 5 Plan

- For breakfast, have an orange juice and blueberry muffin.
- Snack: Dark chocolate chips sprinkled over air-popped popcorn.
- Turkey and avocado wrap for lunch, along with baby carrots and hummus.
- Snack: Raisins and peanut butter on celery sticks
- For dinner, have grilled fish with brown rice and steamed green beans.

Day 6 Plan

- French toast with turkey sausage and pieces of melon for breakfast.

- Bananas with cashew butter as a snack

- Chicken quesadilla with avocado and salsa for lunch

- Snack: Berry-flavored yogurt with honey.

- Quinoa-topped beef and broccoli stir-fry for dinner

Day 7 Plan

- For breakfast, have oatmeal with honey and mixed fruit.

- Snack: Whole grain crackers and cheese

- Lunch: Chicken breast filled with spinach and feta served with roasted veggies.

- Snack: A smoothie made with almond milk and mixed fruit.

- Supper will consist of sweet potato fries and grilled turkey burgers.

CHAPTER 6

Dietary Strategies for Kids with ADHD

Various dietary approaches may benefit ADHD children in addition to lowering sugar consumption and boosting omega-3 fatty acids. To name a few:

1. A Breakfast High in Protein

For children with ADHD, a breakfast high in protein may improve alertness and concentration. Protein boosts mood, gives sustained energy throughout the day, and helps keep blood sugar levels stable. Eggs, Greek yogurt, turkey, chicken, and fish are all excellent sources of protein.

2. Foods High in Magnesium

Magnesium, a necessary mineral that is needed for brain function, has been discovered to be lower in children with ADHD.

Magnesium is included in several foods, including spinach, almonds, pumpkin seeds, and black beans.

3. Fruits and vegetables that is vibrant

According to studies, children with ADHD benefit from eating a diet heavy in colorful fruits and vegetables, especially those that are strong in antioxidants. Antioxidants enhance cognitive performance and protect brain cells from harm. Blueberries, strawberries, and leafy greens like kale and spinach are foods that are especially rich in antioxidants.

4. Stay clear of food additives

Hyperactivity and other behavioral problems in kids with ADHD have been related to food additives such as artificial sweeteners, colors, and preservatives.

ADHD symptoms may be lessened by avoiding processed meals, sweets, drinks, and other sugary snacks.

5. Cut down on dairy and gluten

Gluten or dairy sensitivity may exist in certain ADHD kids. Digestive disorders, allergies, and behavioral challenges may all be brought on by these sensitivities. Some kids' conduct and attentiveness might be improved by decreasing or eliminating certain meals.

Every kid is unique, so what works for one child may not work for another. This is a crucial point to remember. The ideal nutritional approach for your child's unique requirements might be determined by consulting a qualified dietitian or other healthcare professional.

Essential Benefits of Omega-3 fatty acids and Probiotics

- **Fatty Acids omega-3**

The human body greatly benefits from the important polyunsaturated fatty acid class known as omega-3 fatty acids. These necessary fatty acids must come from one's diet since the body is unable to generate them. The three major omega-3 fatty acids eicosapentaenoic acid (EPA), docosahexaenoic acid (DHA), and alpha-linolenic acid are crucial for human health (ALA).

Some of the several advantages of omega-3 fatty acids are listed below:

1. Heart Health: Omega-3 fatty acids are known to enhance heart health by decreasing blood pressure, reducing the danger of blood clots, and reducing the risk of coronary heart disease.

2. DHA, one of the omega-3 fatty acids, is essential for sustaining and developing brain function. In elderly persons, it also aids in lowering the risk of Alzheimer's disease and cognitive decline.

3. Joint Health: Omega-3 fatty acids are a fantastic choice for those with arthritis because of their anti-inflammatory characteristics, which may help lessen joint pain and stiffness.

4. Eye Health: DHA is crucial for eye health and may help lower the incidence of dry eye syndrome and macular degeneration.

5. Skin Health: By lowering inflammation and enhancing the skin's natural moisture barrier, omega-3 fatty acids may aid to promote skin health. Also, it could be beneficial for ailments like eczema and acne.

Probiotics

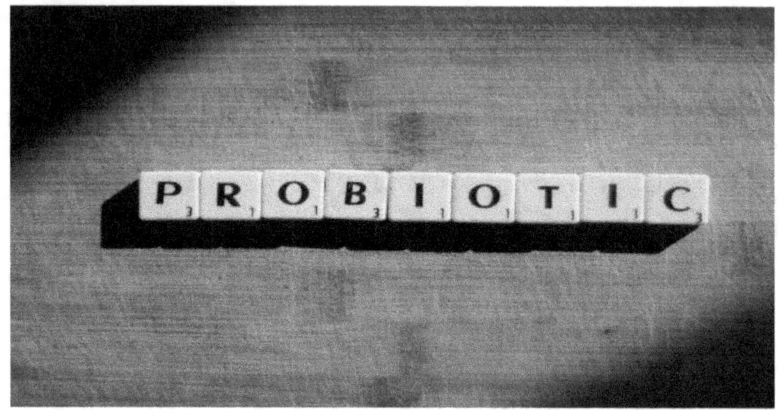

Probiotics are good bacteria that reside in the gut and may support the maintenance of a healthy digestive tract. These beneficial bacteria are necessary for maintaining a balanced gut microbiome and may be found in certain meals and supplements.

These are a few advantages of probiotics:

1. Digestive Health: By boosting the number of good bacteria in the stomach, probiotics may assist to enhance digestive health. This is beneficial for problems including bloating, constipation, and diarrhea.

2. Immune system: Probiotics may strengthen the immune system by boosting antibody production and enhancing gut barrier performance.

3. Mental health: Probiotics may help to boost mood and lessen the symptoms of anxiety and sadness. The gut-brain link is a crucial component of mental health.

4. Probiotics are excellent in lowering the risk of cavities and gum disease.

5. Women's Health: Probiotics may help prevent and cure vaginal infections including yeast infections and bacterial vaginosis, which can be beneficial for women.

Probiotics and omega-3 fatty acids both provide several health advantages that may enhance general well-being. To maintain optimum health, one must consume these nutrients in their diet or think about taking supplements.

The Importance of Hydration for Kids with ADHD

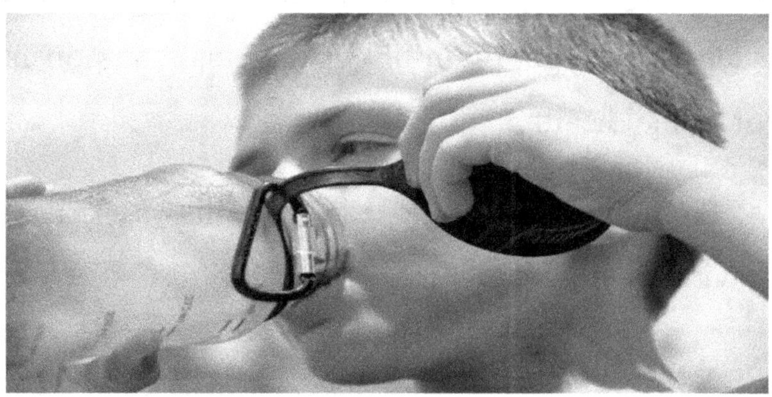

ADHD may be treated in several ways, including through counseling, medication, and dietary modifications. While it may not be the first thing that springs to mind when treating a kid, staying hydrated is essential for their health and well-being, particularly if they have ADHD.

Studies have shown that dehydration has an impact on cognitive performance, emotions, and general physical health. The human brain is about two-thirds water. Since they often fail to drink enough water and might get preoccupied while doing so, children with ADHD are especially prone to dehydration.

Dehydration may make ADHD symptoms worse by causing irritation, lack of focus, and hyperactivity.

For kids with ADHD, drinking water daily is crucial since it may enhance their cognitive ability, and mental clarity, and decrease hyperactivity. Dehydration, according to studies, may impair cognitive function, making it challenging for kids with ADHD to concentrate and complete activities.

Dehydration affects a child's brain function, which causes exhaustion, headaches, and a lack of motivation for chores. To maximize their brain function, it is crucial to make sure that children with ADHD are well-hydrated.

By controlling their mood, children with ADHD may benefit from hydration in another manner. Children may find it difficult to control their emotions due to the irritability and mood changes that may result from dehydration.

Children can better manage their behavior and responses when they are well hydrated, which also helps to regulate mood and emotions. The hormone cortisol, which causes stress and anxiety, may be reduced with regular water consumption, which can promote tranquility, attention, and impulse control.

ADHD often includes symptoms of hyperactivity. Children who have ADHD often have problems sitting still and are restless and fidgety. Hydrating may be very helpful in bringing down hyperactivity. Regular hydration may assist the body cool down and lower its core temperature, which will aid with restlessness and impulse control.

Kids with ADHD need to drink enough water. It may enhance their mental capacity, control their emotions and moods, and even lessen hyperactivity. These advantages not only help kids with ADHD, but they also promote general well-being and excellent health.

To achieve adequate hydration levels, it's crucial to advise kids with ADHD to drink water often, stay away from sugary beverages, and drink water before and after physical activity. A sound hydration strategy may significantly impact a child's mental and emotional well-being, enhancing academic achievement and overall life pleasure.

Strategies for Picky Eaters Kids with ADHD

Having finicky eating habits makes it challenging for parents to provide their ADHD children with a balanced and nourishing diet. Picky eating is a problem that affects a lot of kids, but it may be particularly tough for kids with ADHD since they often struggle with sensory difficulties and having control over their hunger. Parents may, however, use a variety of techniques to persuade their fussy eaters to consume a balanced diet.

1. Establish a Regular Eating Schedule

For ADHD finicky eaters, developing a routinized eating schedule is helpful. Children with ADHD frequently skip meals or eat excessively in one sitting because they find it difficult to control their hunger.

By creating a pattern they can follow, you can prevent them from being overly hungry or full by teaching them when to anticipate meals and snacks. Also, this habit might help you stay more focused and energized all day long.

2. Let your child make decisions

For fussy eaters, giving them some influence over their food might be a good tactic. Offer children a range of wholesome choices, and then nudge them toward the one they like. By empowering the youngster, this method reduces their anxiety about eating and increases their willingness to try new foods. To guarantee a balanced diet, be sure to include a range of meals, such as fruits, vegetables, protein, and carbs.

3. Presentation of Food in a Unique and Colorful Way

When it comes to lunch, presentation is important, particularly for finicky eaters. A meal may be more pleasurable for children with ADHD who often suffer from sensory difficulties if the food is presented colorfully and imaginatively.

Encourage your kid to use fruits, veggies, and other wholesome foods to make their patterns or faces. This will make eating enjoyable and interesting for them.

4. Gently introduce new foods

It might be difficult to introduce new meals to fussy eaters, particularly those with ADHD. It's crucial to begin gradually and include one new dish at a time. Make it enjoyable, include your kid, and involve them in the planning. Urge them to taste it, and then try it again the next day if they don't like it. They could ultimately develop a taste for the new meal if they continue.

5. Be mindful of the texture

Picky eaters often struggle with textures, which may be especially difficult for youngsters with ADHD-related sensory difficulties.

Because of their texture, some youngsters could reject some meals, such as those that are too soft or too crunchy. Try out several textures to discover which ones your youngster prefers. For instance, if kids like crisp dishes and dislike mushy ones, consider roasting veggies or grilling poultry.

6. Give wholesome snacks

For ADHD finicky eaters, providing nutritious snacks throughout the day is essential. By stabilizing blood sugar levels, these foods might lessen the likelihood of mood swings and hyperactivity. Variety is key, so provide sliced fruits and veggies, nuts, seeds, and hummus, among other things. For the snack to keep your youngster feeling full and content, try to include protein.

It might be challenging to feed fussy eaters with ADHD, but with the appropriate approaches and perseverance, it is possible to provide a nutritious and balanced diet. It all comes down to knowing what works for your kid and implementing a regular schedule that encourages creativity and variation. Together, parents and kids may break the cycle of fussy eating and enhance their general health and well-being.

CHAPTER 7

How to Manage Eating Difficulties in Kids

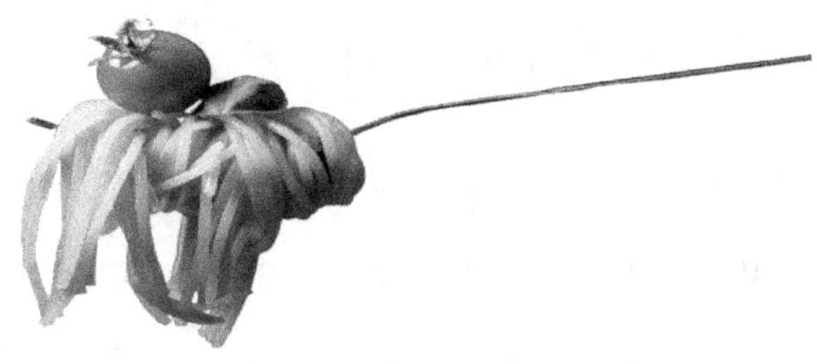

Children often have eating problems, which may be tough for parents to deal with. Some children may act out, refuse to eat, or have sensory difficulties that make trying new meals difficult. To make sure that your child continues to eat a balanced diet, you must address these challenges. The following techniques may be used to control children's eating issues:

1. Provide a welcoming dining atmosphere

A child's dining environment may have a big influence on their eating habits. Set up a relaxing and comfortable dining area to make mealtime enjoyable for your child.

Disconnect the TV and other electronics so that your youngster can concentrate on eating. Make sure there are no distractions and that the table is properly placed.

2. Provide a range of meal options

Your child's diet must include different foods if you want to help them develop a broader palette. Provide a range of foods, such as fresh produce, whole grains, lean protein, and fruits and vegetables.

To avoid overloading your youngster, it's important to introduce new foods gradually and in tiny doses. To make food more appetizing, consider serving it in a variety of ways, such as cooked or raw.

3. Establish regular mealtimes

Your youngster may build a schedule and avoid nibbling throughout the day by having set mealtimes. Make sure your kid eats three meals a day, including any required snacks in between. By doing this, you can control your child's appetite and keep them from overeating or under eating.

4. Include your youngster in the preparation of meals

To get your kid excited about tasting new foods, include them in the planning and preparation of meals. Include your youngster in selecting a dish, chopping up ingredients, or setting the table. They may be more inclined to consume the meal they assisted in preparing if they feel involved and appreciated as a result.

5. Employ reiterative language

While treating eating issues, attempt to employ positive reinforcement as opposed to negative reinforcement. Praising your youngster for trying a new cuisine or activity might inspire them to keep going. A bad connection with food may be cultivated by not using food as a reward or punishment.

6. Consult a professional

Ask a trained therapist, nutritionist, or doctor for assistance if your child's feeding issues continue. They may evaluate your child's nutrition and provide solutions suited to their requirements. To avoid long-term effects, it is important to treat eating disorders as soon as they arise.

Children's eating issues demand persistence, inventiveness, and patience to manage. You can support your child in maintaining a healthy and enjoyable relationship with food by fostering a positive eating environment, providing a variety of food options, establishing regular mealtimes, involving your child in meal preparation, using positive reinforcement, and getting professional assistance.

Effect of Sensory Processing Disorder on kids ADHD

A child's intellectual, social, and emotional development may be greatly impacted by ADHD, which often results in subpar academic performance, behavioral issues, and social isolation.

Sensory Processing Disorder (SPD), which affects how a person reacts to sensory information and causes problems processing and regulating sensory input, is another disorder that often co-occurs with ADHD. The functioning of a kid may be significantly impacted by SPD, which can exacerbate the signs of ADHD.

ADHD and Sensory Processing

How the brain receives, decodes, and reacts to sensory information from the environment is referred to as " sensory processing." The majority of people naturally analyze sensory information and utilize it to generate appropriate reactions.

Yet, sensory information may be interpreted differently in children with SPD, leading to over reactive or under-reactive behaviors. Many sensory modalities, including touch, hearing, taste, smell, and visual input, may be challenging for kids with SPD.

Sensory processing issues may occur in children with ADHD, but the frequency and severity of these issues might vary. Children who have ADHD may have issues with sensory discrimination, sensory over- or under-response, or both. For instance, individuals could have trouble differentiating between important and irrelevant sensory information or be too sensitive to noise, which makes them easily distracted.

Also, kids with ADHD can look for sensory stimulation to help them self-stimulate, which can result in actions like fidgeting and impulsive conduct.

How SPD can Make ADHD Symptoms Worse

It may be difficult for kids with ADHD to control their actions, emotions, and concentration due to sensory processing issues.

Sensory stimulation may easily divert children with SPD, making it difficult for them to maintain focus and finish activities. Moreover, kids with SPD may struggle to control their reactions to sensory input, which may cause either over- or under-reactivity.

For instance, a kid with ADHD who is very distracted agitated, and challenging to calm down when touched may have touch sensitivity. Moreover, social connections may be impacted by SPD, which can cause social isolation and feelings of rejection in kids. Social signals, such as understanding body language, tone of voice, and facial expressions, may be challenging for kids with SPD.

They could also have issues with physical contact and nonverbal communication, which can cause misunderstandings and misinterpretations.

However, a kid with SPD may experience anxiety, despair, and poor self-esteem due to its impact on their mental health. Children with SPD may experience tension and anxiety as a result of feeling over stimulated by sensory stimulation. Along with feeling different from their classmates or misunderstood, children with ADHD and SPD may experience feelings of loneliness and poor self-worth.

Intervention

Children with ADHD and SPD may benefit greatly from early intervention in terms of improved functioning and quality of life. Children with SPD are often given occupational therapy as a main intervention, with an emphasis on sensory integration methods that are meant to help a kid better integrate and regulate sensory information.

A child's fine and gross motor abilities, visual-perceptual abilities, and self-control may all be enhanced with occupational therapy.

Finally, SPD may have a substantial negative effect on a child's functioning, aggravating the signs of ADHD. Children with ADHD and SPD may struggle with paying attention, interacting with others, and feeling emotionally safe, which may hurt academic achievement, behavioral issues, and social isolation. The functionality and quality of life of a child may be improved by early intervention, such as occupational therapy.

Mealtime Behavior on Kids ADHD

Children with ADHD may have a variety of difficulties throughout the day, including issues with eating. As compared to children who are usually growing, they often exhibit atypical eating behaviors, which may affect their development, nutrition, and general health.

A child's conduct at meals, such as sitting still, paying attention, taking turns, and adhering to food-related norms, is referred to as mealtime behavior. Given that children with ADHD sometimes struggle to sit still or remain focused for lengthy periods, poor conduct during meals may be a big issue for parents and other adults who are responsible for them.

Due of the heightened sensory input from the textures, scents, tastes, and social interaction of food during mealtime, this behavior may become more obvious. The following are some typical eating habits of children with ADHD:

1. Food avoidance: Children with ADHD may find it difficult to experiment with novel tastes or textures, which results in a lack of food options and poor nutrition.

2. Impulsivity: Children with ADHD could grab, taste, or touch various meals without asking first, wasting food and posing safety risks.

3. Hyperactivity: Children with ADHD may fidget or wriggle while eating, causing accidents, messes, and even injury.

4. Distractibility: Kids with ADHD are more likely to become easily distracted during meals, which may result in missed signals, incomplete meals, and social disengagement.

5. Lack of social skills: Children with ADHD may find it difficult to follow social signals and take turns at meals, which may cause disputes and social isolation.

Parents and caregivers may use a variety of techniques to address these issues with mealtime behavior, including:

1. Create clear rules and expectations: Setting clear rules and expectations for meals may assist children with ADHD understand what is expected of them, such as sitting still, using utensils, tasting new foods, and taking turns.

2. Provide children with ADHD structure and routine by establishing regular meal and snack times. This will help the kids get ready for and look forward to meals.

3. Employ positive reinforcement to encourage children to behave better and develop more favorable attitudes about food. Praise kids for excellent mealtime conduct, such as trying new foods or adhering to rules.

4. Provide sensory input: Giving children with ADHD sensory input during meals, such as letting them sample foods or using a weighted lap cushion, may help them settle down and concentrate.

5. Include the child in meal preparation: Getting kids involved in meal preparation activities like cooking or grocery shopping may spur their interest in trying new foods and enhance their eating manners.

The way a kid behaves at meals has a significant impact on their physical, social, and emotional well-being throughout the day. Mealtime behavior may be especially difficult for kids with ADHD, necessitating a range of tactics from parents and caregivers to encourage healthy eating and good behaviors.

Parents and other adults who care for children with ADHD may assist these kids in forming good eating habits that will serve them well throughout their lives by being aware of their particular requirements.

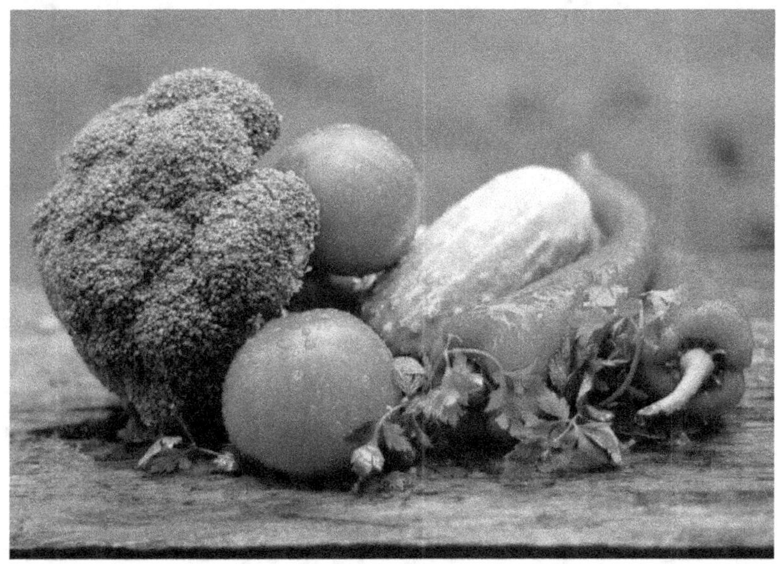

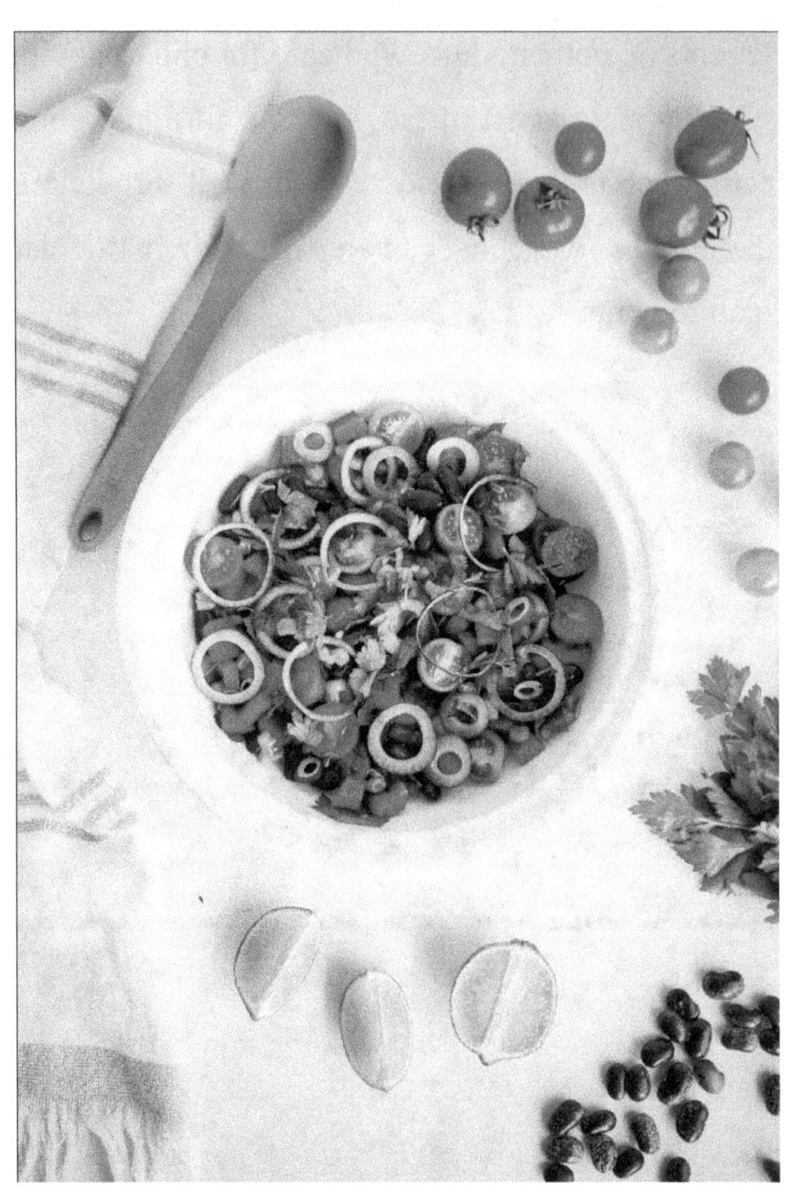

CHAPTER 8

Creating Sustainable and Healthy Eating Habits for ADHD Children

Research suggests that food and nutrition are important in treating ADHD in kids. It is possible to provide vital nutrients that support brain growth, control mood, and enhance focus by developing enduring and healthy eating habits. In this post, we'll look at some advice for helping kids with ADHD develop enduring and good eating habits.

1. Prioritize balanced meals

A balanced diet with all the necessary nutrients is necessary for children with ADHD to improve brain function and encourage healthy development. A balanced lunch should include a variety of fruits and vegetables, proteins, healthy fats, and carbs.

Proteins are needed to create and repair tissues, healthy fats help with brain growth, and carbohydrates provide the brain with the energy it needs to function.

2. Don't eat processed foods

The symptoms of ADHD might increase because processed meals are often heavy in sugar, salt, and harmful fats. According to studies, people with ADHD are less tolerant of processed meals and more susceptible to their negative consequences. Thus, it's essential to stay away from processed meals like fast food, sweets, and soda.

3. Put Whole Foods First

Whole foods are those that have undergone little or no processing and yet contain all of their original nutrients.

Healthy meals provide the vital nutrients required for a healthy brain's growth and may assist regulate blood sugar levels, which can enhance attention and concentration.

4. Limit Your Sugar Consumption

In children with ADHD, high sugar consumption has been associated with an increase in restlessness, irritability, and hyperactivity. Thus, it's crucial to cut down on sugar consumption and choose healthy options like fruits, honey, or maple syrup. Sugary foods and beverages like soda and sweets should only be consumed on special occasions.

5. Promote Consistent Meals

Frequent meals provide greater concentration and focus while stabilizing blood sugar levels.

To maintain a constant level of energy throughout the day, children with ADHD should consume breakfast and snacks often. Skipping meals or snacks might make you grumpy, exhausted, and your symptoms of ADHD may become worse.

ADHD Diet and the School Environment

Here are some suggestions for parents and teachers on how to provide a supportive atmosphere for kids with ADHD at school:

1. Consistent Routines: Children with ADHD benefit from structure and regularity. They may keep on track by establishing a dependable routine with precise expectations and timetables.

2. Balanced meals: Eating a healthy, well-balanced diet will help minimize ADHD symptoms by balancing mood and energy levels.

3. Snacks: Provide wholesome snacks throughout the day to assist maintain energy levels and stop meltdowns brought on by hunger.

4. Breaks: Taking regular pauses might assist kids with ADHD maintain their attention and concentration. Exercise or movement for brief intervals may be extremely beneficial.

5. Quiet area: Provide a place where kids may work quietly, read, or take breaks as necessary. Earplugs or headphones with noise cancellation are also beneficial.

6. Positive reinforcement: Giving kids with ADHD positive rewards might encourage them to remain on topic and finish their work.

7. Allowances: Take into account allowances like more time for exams or assignments, preferred seats, or organizational technology.

Overall, fostering a controlled and encouraging learning environment in the classroom may help individuals with ADHD flourish socially and intellectually.

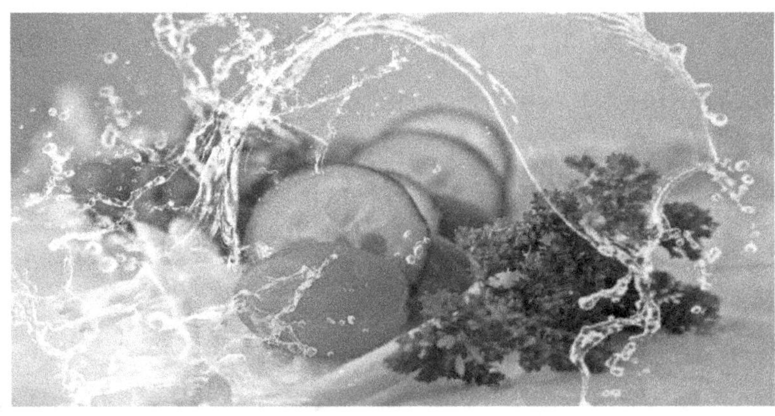

CONCLUSION

An ADHD diet for children may make a substantial difference in how well ADHD symptoms like impulsivity, hyperactivity, and inattention are managed. Every kid is different; therefore what may work for one child may not necessarily work for another. This is an important concept to grasp.

Yet, research indicates that removing processed meals, sugary snacks, and artificial colors and tastes from a child's diet may greatly lessen the symptoms of ADHD. Instead, eating a diet high in whole foods, such as fruits, vegetables, lean meats, and healthy fats, may provide you with the nutrients you need for good mental health and encourage good conduct.

For kids with ADHD, it's important to drink enough water, engage in regular exercise, and get adequate sleep in addition to eating a balanced diet. To provide a supportive and caring environment that takes into account all facets of a child's health and well-being, parents and other caregivers must collaborate.

It is important to remember that managing ADHD symptoms may need more than just good eating. Depending on the severity of the problem, behavioral therapy, medications, and other interventions may also be required. Yet, including a balanced diet in a child's daily routine may help manage ADHD symptoms and advance general health and well-being.

In the end, parents and other adults who are responsible for a kid with ADHD should seek advice from a healthcare expert to decide the best course of action. Even if their kid has been diagnosed with ADHD, parents, and caregivers may support their child's success by working together to execute an extensive treatment plan.

For kids with ADHD, the appropriate nutrition may make all the difference. Lean proteins, whole grains, and leafy greens are healthy meal choices that may aid with attention, control hyperactivity, and general cognitive performance. Remember that although a nutritious diet won't magically cure ADHD, it may surely help your kid live a fuller, healthier life. Hence, let's place a high priority on nutritious nutrition to offer our children the greatest opportunity to flourish.

Dear Parent,

I am aware that finding out your kid has been diagnosed with ADHD may be a trying and stressful situation. However, I want to offer you a letter of hope and encouragement today.

First, understand that you're not on your own. Worldwide, both children and adults are impacted by the illness known as ADHD. From support groups to counseling services to educational materials, there are innumerable tools available to assist you and your kid get through this journey.

Second, having ADHD does not automatically condemn one to a lifetime of suffering. Even though there is no cure for ADHD, there are several interventions and therapies that may support your child's development and help them manage their symptoms.

Children with ADHD are capable of leading fulfilling lives with the correct assistance.

When you go with your kid on this trip, bear the following in mind:

- The importance of early diagnosis and treatment. The earlier you identify and treat your child's ADHD, the simpler it will be to control their symptoms and stop any unfavorable effects from their conduct.

- Learn about ADHD along with your kid. You will be better prepared to handle its problems the more you understand about this condition. To understand more about ADHD and its treatments, there are a ton of books, websites, and other resources accessible.

- Create a specialized treatment plan with the help of your child's doctor. Working closely with your kid's doctor or therapist to create a plan that works best for them is essential since treatment for ADHD differs based on the requirements of each unique child. This might include a mix of treatment, medication, behavioral interventions, or all of the above.

- Pay attention to your child's abilities rather than their shortcomings. Children with ADHD often exhibit special skills and abilities, such as creativity, curiosity, and a love of learning. Encourage your kid to follow their passions and engage in things that make them happy and fulfilled.

- Honor your child's accomplishments, no matter how tiny. There will probably be ups and downs along the process of managing

ADHD. Take the time to recognize your child's accomplishments and rejoice in every tiny win.

I'd want to end by saying that you are a wonderful parent and should be proud of yourself. You are providing the greatest care for your kid, which is difficult to do while dealing with an ADHD diagnosis. Your kid may learn to control their symptoms and grow with commitment, tolerance, and optimism.

If you need help in aiding your child's recovery or you need someone to talk to, I'm always a message away via diettalkwithelisa@yahoo.com

Best wishes,

Elisa T. Morrison

Bonus: 4 Weeks Meal Planner for Kids

WEEK ONE

	BREAKFAST	LUNCH	DINNER
MON			
TUES			
WED			
THURS			
FRI			
SAT			
SUN			

WEEK TWO

	BREAKFAST	LUNCH	DINNER
MON			
TUES			
WED			
THURS			
FRI			
SAT			
SUN			

WEEK THREE

	BREAKFAST	LUNCH	DINNER
MON			
TUES			
WED			
THURS			
FRI			
SAT			
SUN			

WEEK FOUR

	BREAKFAST	LUNCH	DINNER
MON			
TUES			
WED			
THURS			
FRI			
SAT			
SUN